ANNA

and her
RAINBOW-COLORED
yoga mats

By Giselle Shardlow

Illustrated by Paul Wrangles

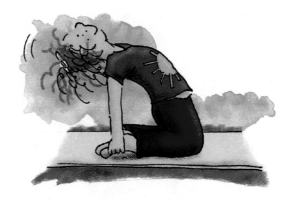

Anna and her Rainbow-Colored Yoga Mats

Copyright © 2014 by Giselle Shardlow

Cover and illustrations by Paul Wrangles
All images © 2012 Giselle Shardlow

Second Edition

ISBN-13: 978-1477400777

ISBN-10: 147740077X

www.kidsyogastories.com

Email us at info@kidsyogastories.com

What do you think?

Let us know what you think of
Anna and her Rainbow-Colored Yoga Mats
at feedback@kidsyogastories.com.

Printed in the U.S.A.

For my mum and dad,
who always encourage me to follow my dreams

~ G.S. ~

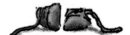

To my wife (and encourager) Ruth

~ P.W. ~

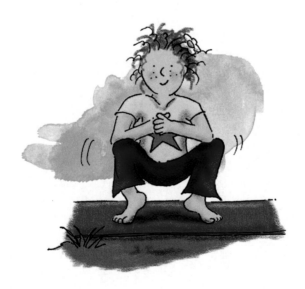

Foreword

I am excited to have been asked to write the foreword for this beautiful book written by my dear friend, Giselle Shardlow. Giselle is a mother, a yogini, a teacher, and one of the most thoughtful, kind, and fun-loving people I know. All of this comes through in her writing for children.

Giselle encourages children to think of others, to celebrate diversity, and to move their bodies without feeling self-conscious or competitive. Children these days are under more pressure than ever. They feel the sense of competition and pressure to succeed as much as adults. Like adults, children often internalize this stress and do not necessarily express their emotions. However their stress may come out in frustration, anxiety, and even conditions such as asthma and eczema. Yoga teaches children to breathe, to relax, to let go, and to step off the treadmill of competition. It can offer valuable techniques for stressful situations and give children tools for conflict resolution, preparing for exams, managing peer-pressure, and making good choices. Introducing yoga to young children gives them a valuable foundation for life, a foundation of love, fun, and creativity.

Reading is one of the most powerful and positive experiences you and your children can do together. Some of my own happiest memories are of my mother reading stories to me as a child. Now that I am a mother myself, some of the deepest moments of peace and connection I have with my sons are when we are reading together. Reading a book with your child can be the springboard for dialogues about all kinds of different topics which may be difficult to discuss or open up without a context. The activities in Giselle's book do not require special equipment, and they are free!

My sons and I have really enjoyed this storybook.
We hope that you enjoy it as well.

Katie Manitsas
Director of Jivamukti Yoga Sydney
Author of *Yoga Off the Mat* and *The Yoga of Birth*

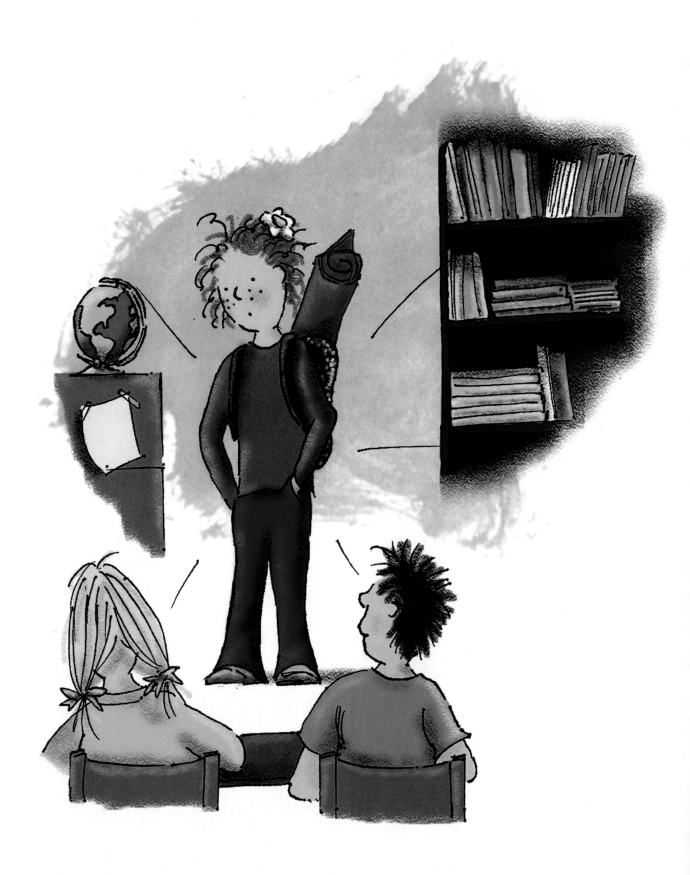

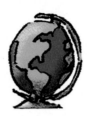

"Say hello to Anna," announced the teacher.
"She's our new student from the country."

Anna looked down at her toes.
She felt a pain in her stomach.

"HELLO, AAAANNAAA!" chimed the class.

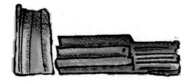

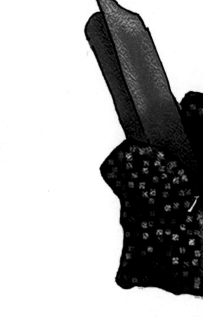

"What is that red thing
in her sparkly backpack?"

"Check out her curly hair!"

"Look at her crazy-colored shoes!"
whispered the children to each other.

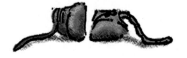

Anna couldn't hear them.

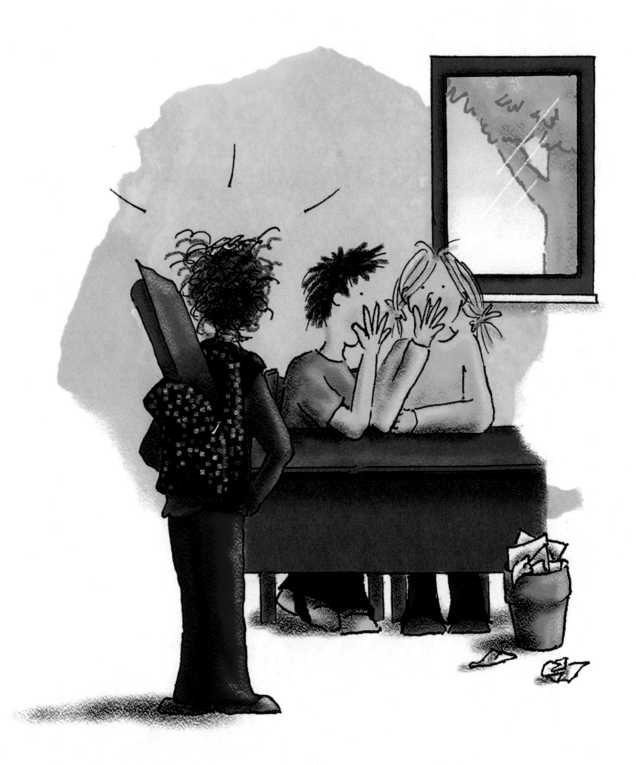

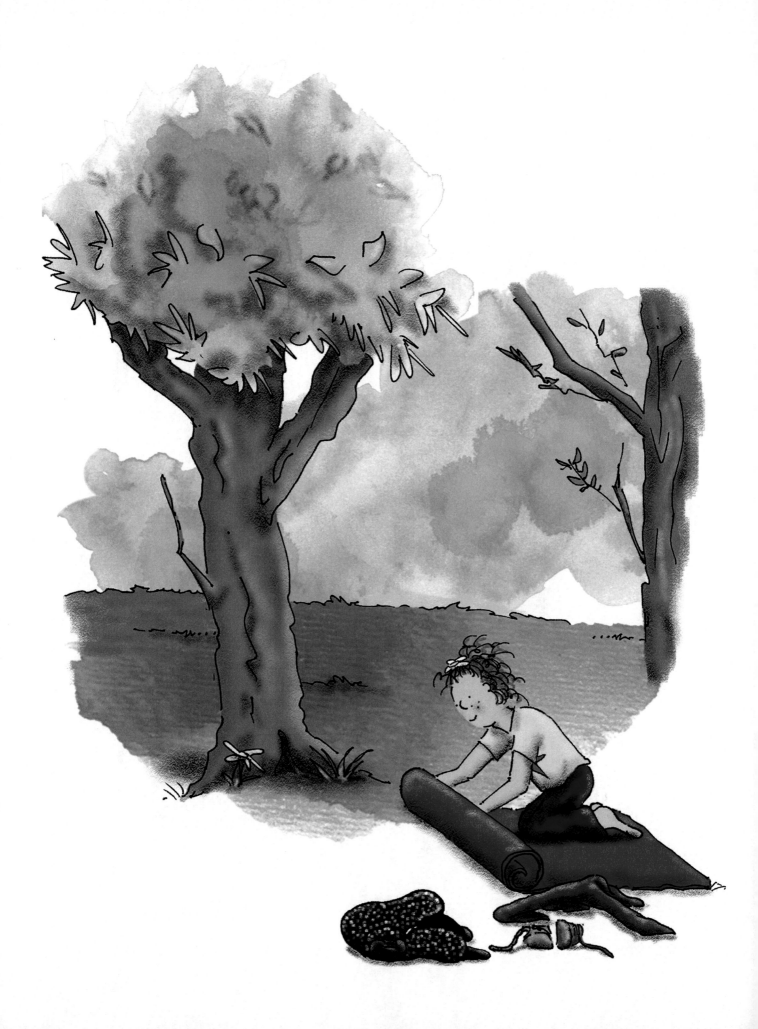

At recess, Anna unrolled
her red yoga mat next to the tree.

She felt safe on her yoga mat.

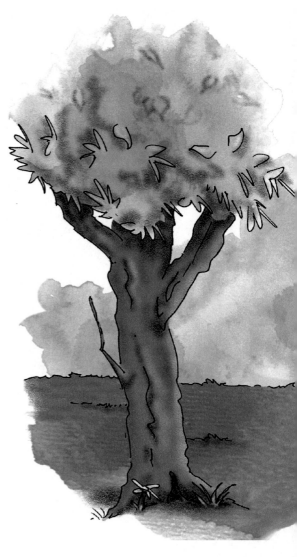

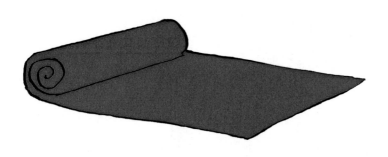

She had learned to do yoga
by watching her mom
every morning.

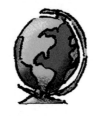

As she moved
through her poses,
she imagined traveling the world.

That day,
Anna imagined going on a farm adventure.

She arched up like a cat.

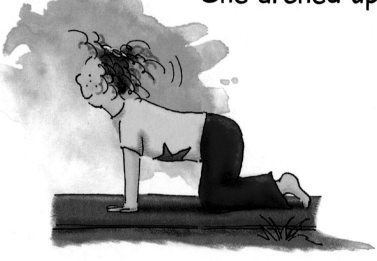

She kicked up like a horse...

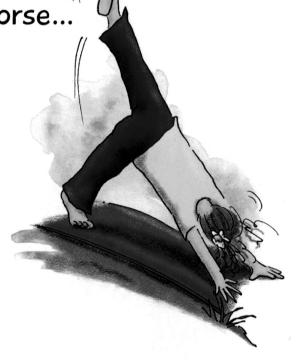

and she waddled like a duck.

Anna was in her own little world
on her red yoga mat.

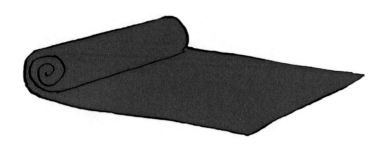

She couldn't hear the five children watching her.

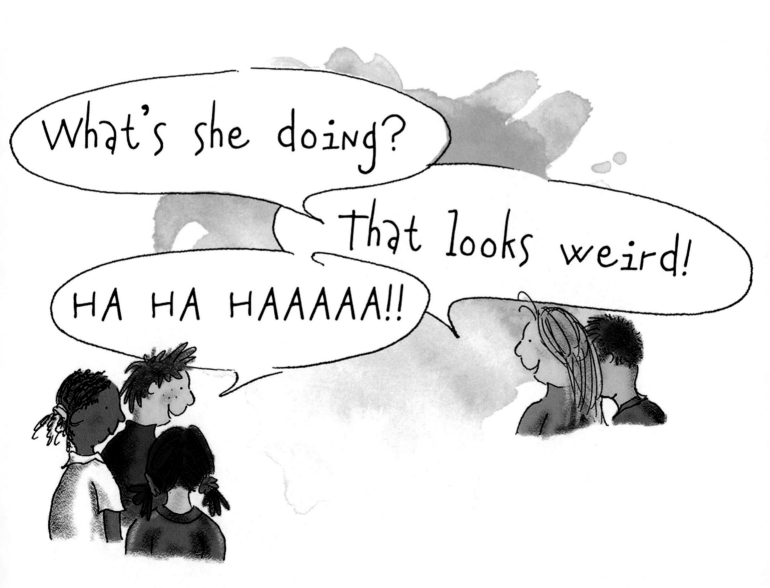

What's she doing?

that looks weird!

HA HA HAAAAA!!

The next day, at recess,
Anna unrolled her orange yoga mat next to the tree.

That day she imagined
a journey to the jungle.

She swayed like a palm tree.

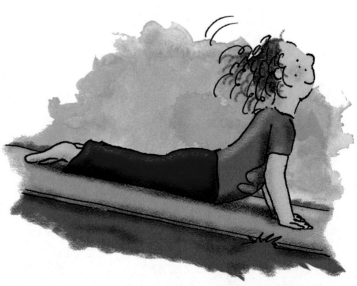

She stretched
like a jaguar...

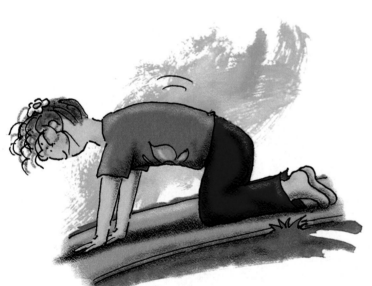

and she hissed
like a snake.

Anna was in her own little world
on her orange yoga mat.

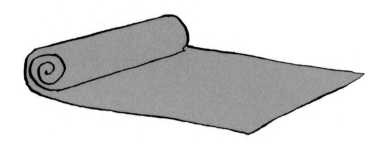

She couldn't hear the ten children watching her.

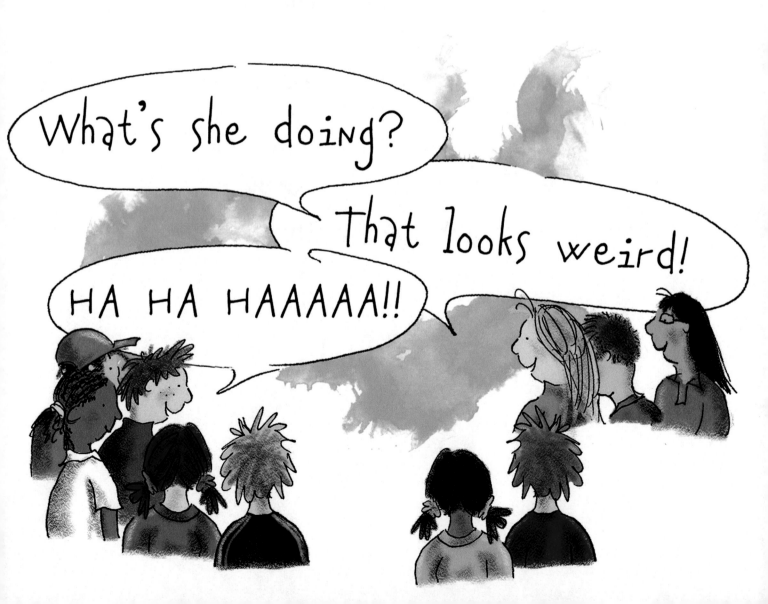

Anna looked forward to recess time.
She ignored the funny looks and laughter
from the other children.

Her mother always said to her,

"Be true to yourself, Anna.
If you want to be happy,

then you must be happy for others around you."

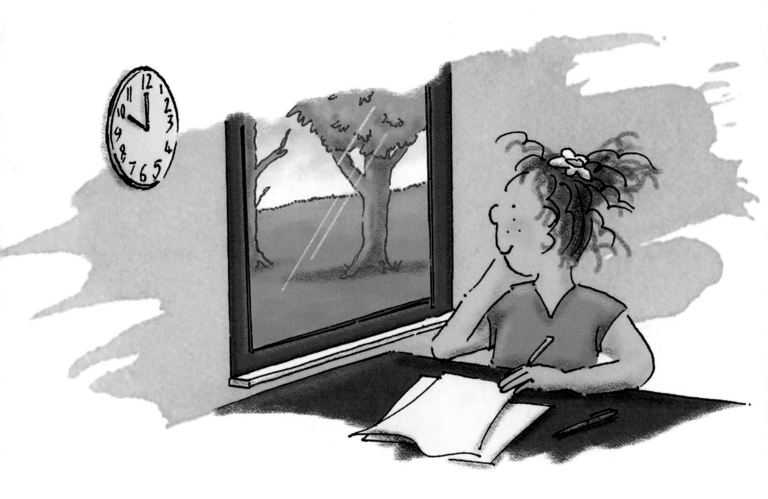

Every day, she remembered what her mother said.
She thought about being happy inside.
She tried not to worry that she didn't fit in
or that she was different.

The following day,
Anna unrolled her yellow yoga mat next to the tree.

That day she imagined a safari to the desert.

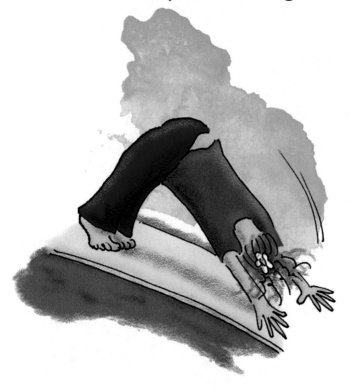

She stretched up
like a pyramid.

She perched
like a sphinx...

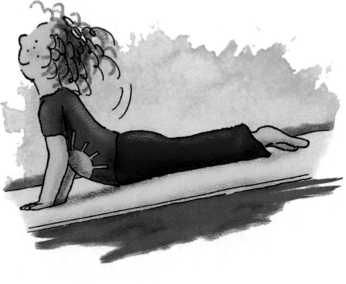

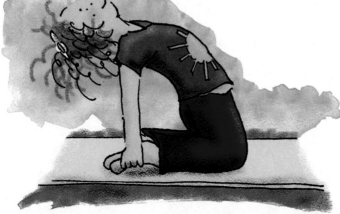

and she bent back
like a camel.

Anna was in her own little world
on her yellow yoga mat.

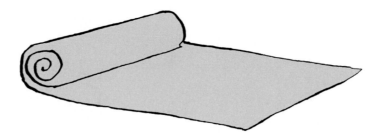

She couldn't hear the twenty children watching her.

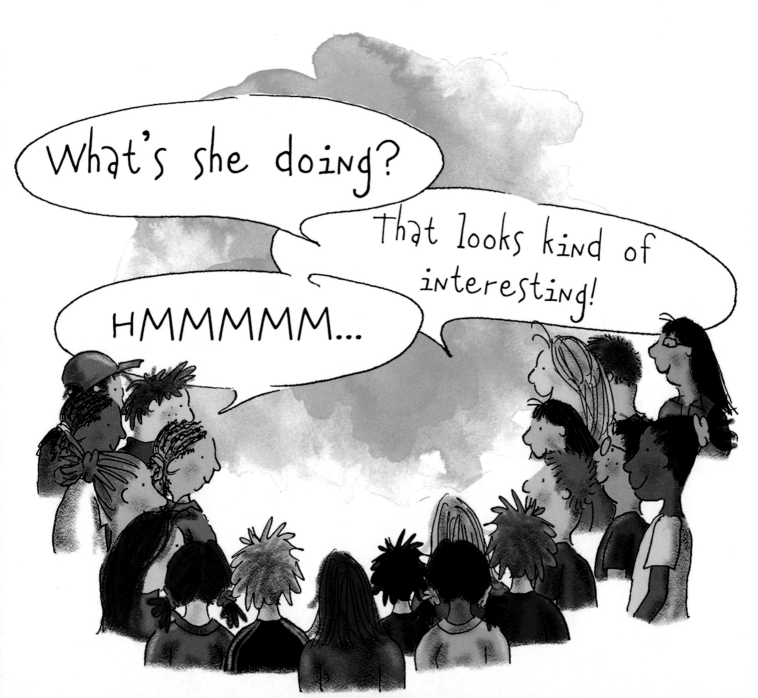

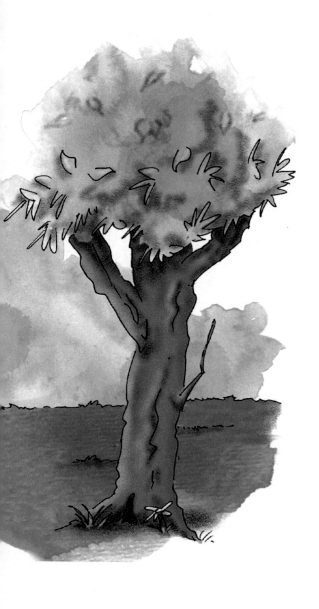

One day,
as Anna was unrolling
her green yoga mat
under the tree,
she felt a soft tap
on her shoulder.

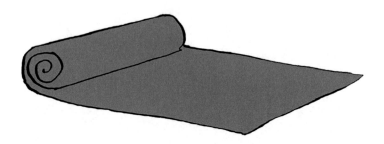

"I have a hearing loss too."
Nick pointed shyly at Anna's hearing aids.

Anna was surprised that Nick was talking to her.
She had noticed groups of giggling girls
following him around the playground.

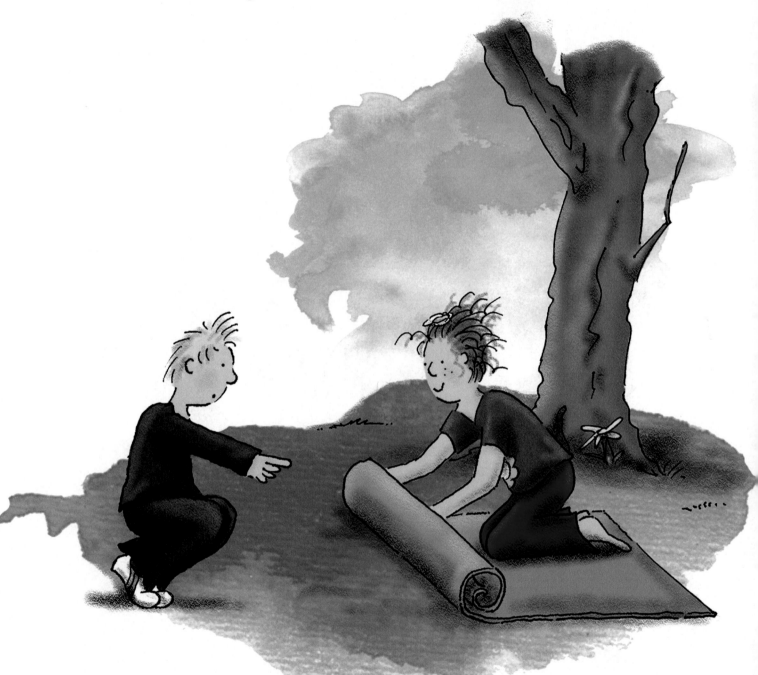

"I lip read. I don't know anyone like me."
Nick pointed to her mat.
"What is it you're doing anyway?"

"I imagine that I am traveling the world. I visit deserts, oceans, and forests." Anna leaped around her mat.

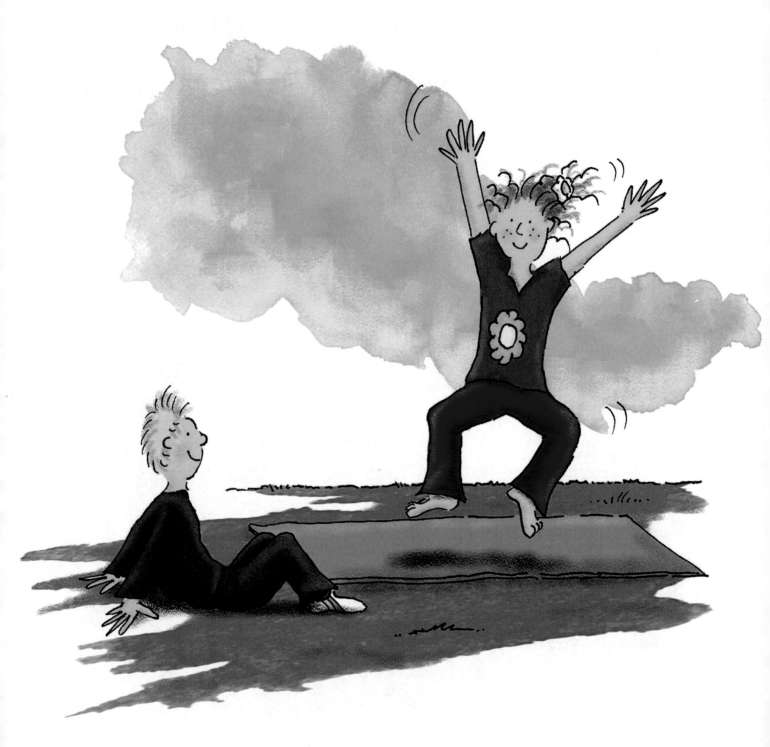

"Why don't I teach you to lip read and you teach me to travel the world?" Nick grinned from ear to ear and felt happy for the first time in a long time.

Each day,
Anna and Nick practiced lip reading together.

And at recess time,
Anna taught Nick how to
travel the world.

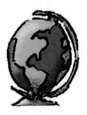

"All you need is a little concentration
and a whole lot of imagination!"
Anna told her new friend.

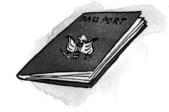

Anna unrolled her blue yoga mat under the tree.
She gave Nick her red one.

They trekked through
the mountains.

They swayed like trees.

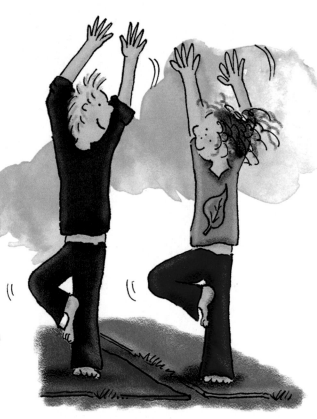

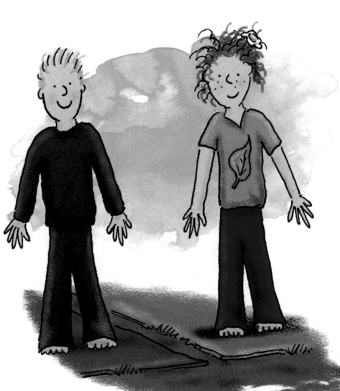

They stood tall
like mountains...

and they moved
like bears.

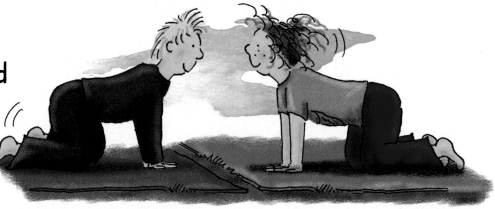

They didn't notice
the group of forty children
watching them.

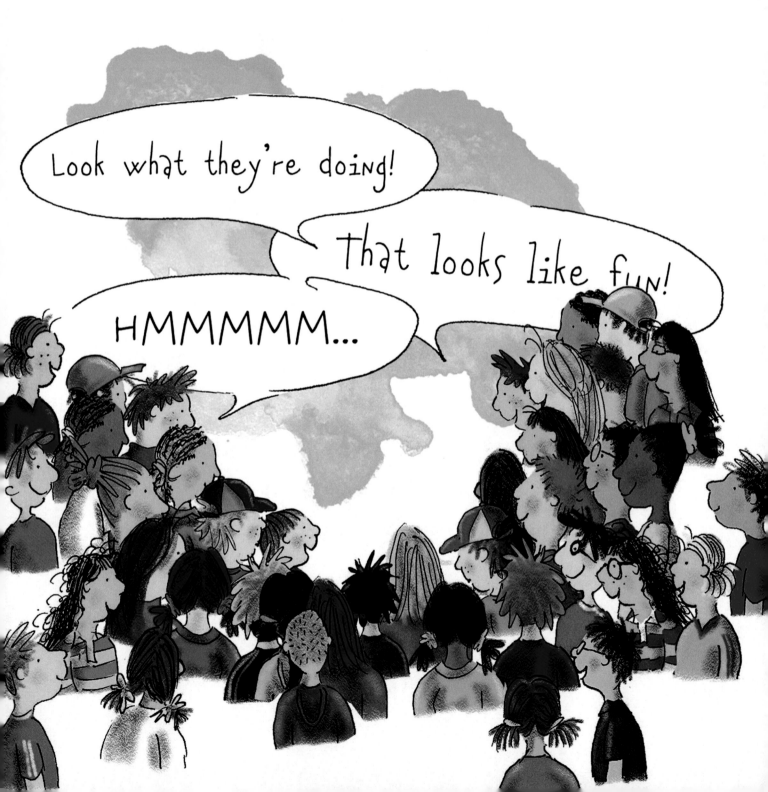

One day, Anna unrolled
her purple yoga mat next to the tree.

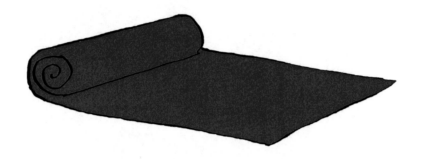

"Let's imagine going to the ocean!"
Nick joined Anna under the tree.

They flapped like swimmers.
They balanced like surfers ...
and they tilted like sails in the wind.

They were so busy being seagulls, sandcastles, and
seashells that they didn't notice the forty children
around them. Suddenly it started to sprinkle.

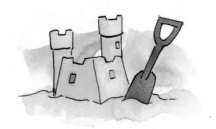

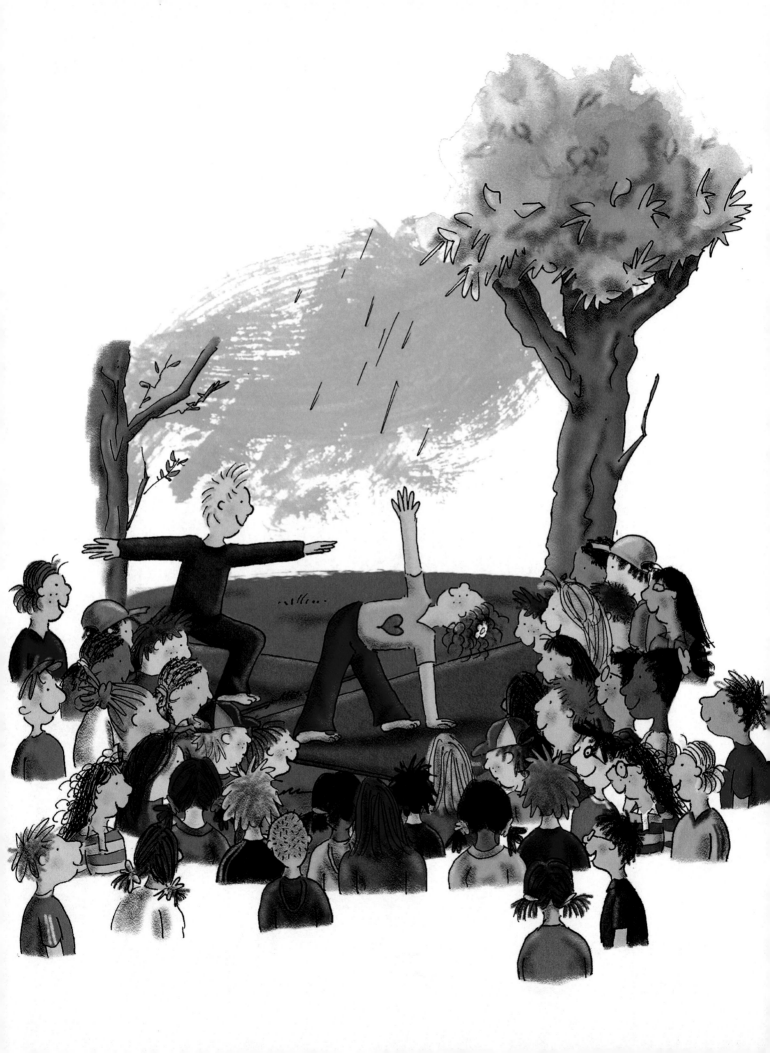

Anna's legs shot up like water from a dolphin's blowhole.
The rain fell gently on her face.
"I'm happy inside and
my dreams have come true!"

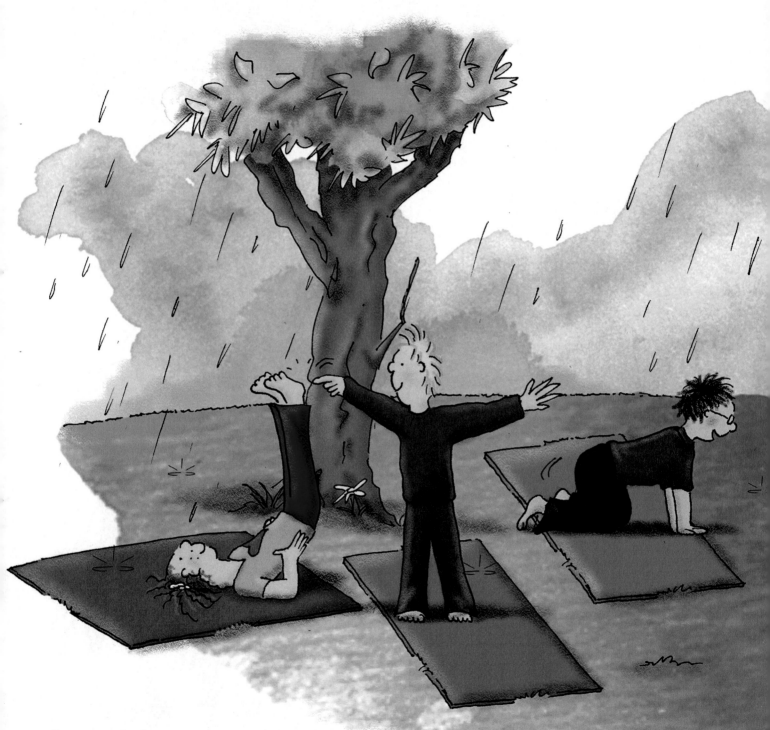

Anna felt a soft tap on her toes.
"Look Anna! Our RAINBOW!" said Nick excitedly.

Anna smiled when she saw that a group of children had come to join them on their own colorful yoga mats.

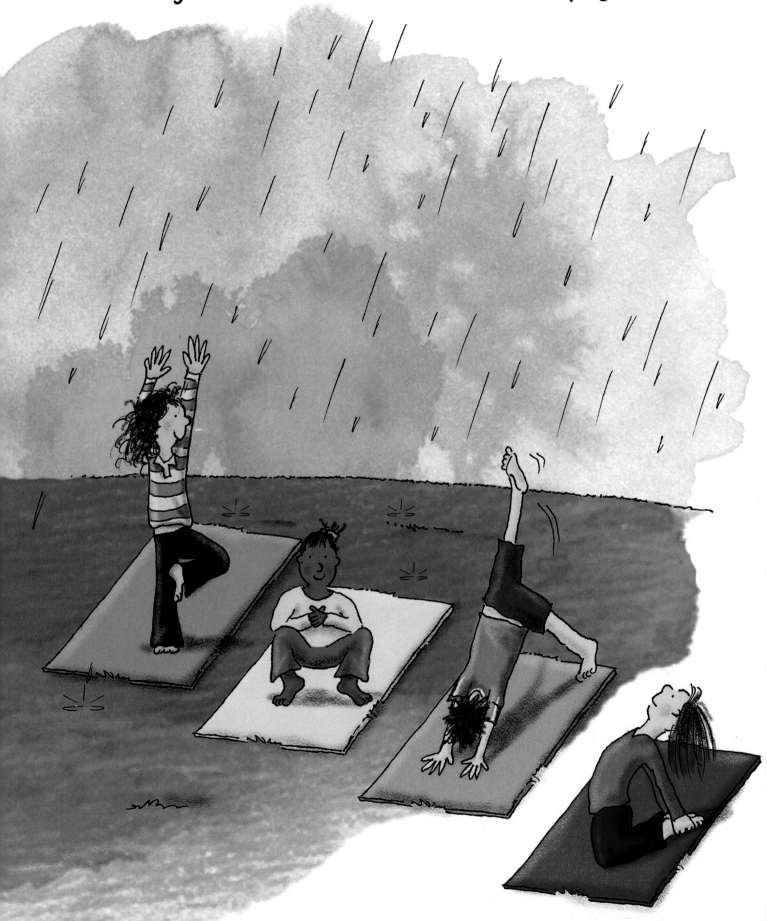

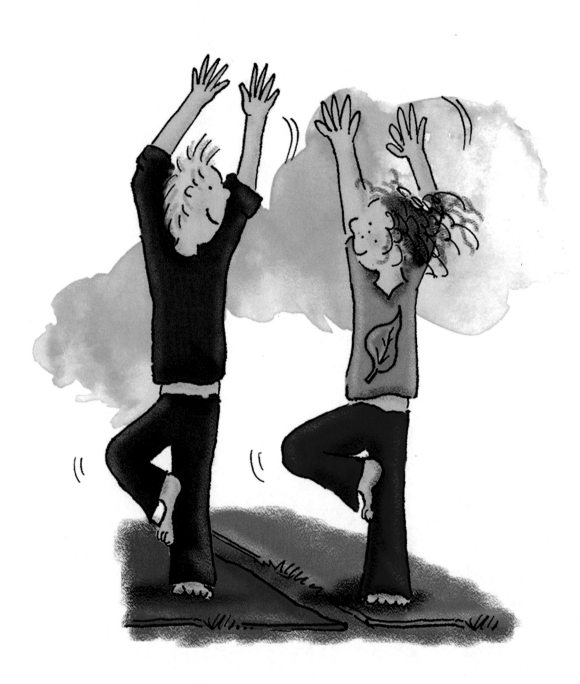

About the Author

Giselle Shardlow hopes to inspire children by drawing from her experiences as an international primary school teacher, world traveler, mother, and yogi. She lives in Boston with her husband and daughter. Her books and other creative resources can be found at www.kidsyogastories.com.

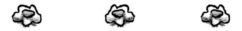

About the Illustrator

Paul Wrangles is a writer and illustrator from South Wales (U.K.). His whimsical illustrations can be found in children's books such as *Matthew and the Wellington Boots* and *The Champion Hare*.

Other Yoga Books
by Giselle Shardlow

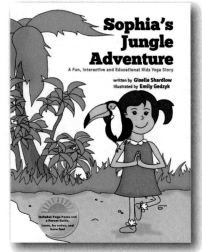

Sophia's Jungle
Adventure

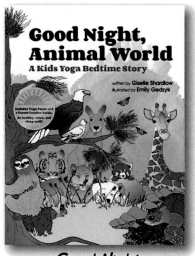

Good Night,
Animal World

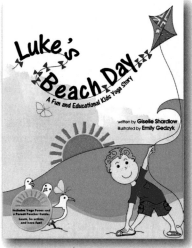

Luke's Beach Day

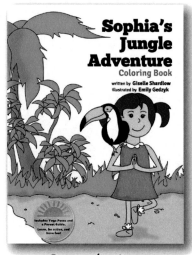

Sophia's Jungle
Adventure
Coloring Book

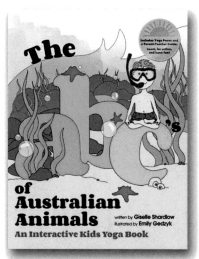

The ABC's of
Australian Animals

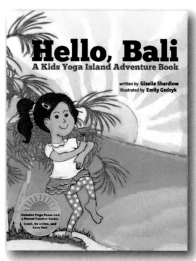

Hello, Bali

Many of the books above are available in
Spanish and eBook format.

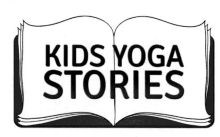

KIDS YOGA
STORIES

www.kidsyogastories.com

Made in the USA
Middletown, DE
20 September 2015